HOW TO CONTROL ALCOHOLISM

PROVEN TECHNIQUES FOR ALCOHOL ABUSE, OVERCOME DEPENDENCY, BREAK ADDICTION AND RECOVER YOUR LIFE

I0407717

BY SMART READS

Free Audiobook

As a thank you for being a Smart Reader you can choose 2 FREE audiobooks from audible.com. Simply sign up for free by visiting www.audibletrial.com/Travis to get your books.

Visit:

www.smartreads.co/freebooks
to receive Smart Reads books for FREE

Check us out on Instagram:

www.instagram.com/smart_readers
@smart_readers

ABOUT SMARTREADS

Choose Smart Reads and get smart every time. Smart Reads sorts through all the best content and condenses the most helpful information into easily digestible chunks.

We design our books to be short, easy to read and highly informative. Leaving you with maximum understanding in the least amount of time.

Smart Reads aims to accelerate the spread of quality information so we've taken the copyright off everything we publish and donate our material directly to the public domain. You can read our uncopyright below.

We believe in paying it forward and donate 5% of our net sales to Pencils of Promise to build schools, train teachers and support child education.

To limit our footprint and restore forests around the globe we are planting a tree for every 10 hardcover books we sell.

Thanks for choosing Smart Reads and helping us help the planet.

Sincerely,

Travis & the Smart Reads Team

TABLE OF CONTENTS

INTRODUCTION

Welcome to How To Set Yourself Free From Alcohol, a book crammed with easy to implement strategies and proven tips to help people quit drinking and live a fulfilling life away from the bottle.

I know you want to quit the booze. I know you want to be ruthless about this. But are you ready? If you're not sure how ready you are to quit right now, it is my hope that by the end of this book you will be totally ready. Indeed, before you finish the book, you might have already taken the first steps to living a cleaner, healthier, better life free from alcohol.

Why quit?

Without alcohol, you get to do so much more. You feel 100% better, look 100% better, and you waste no time living the life you've always dreamed of living. It's like the great investor Warren Buffet said, we all have a weakest link that stops us from living the life we really want, and for many of us that weakest link is alcohol. Here are a few more reasons to give up drinking:

- You will have more cash
- Your thinking will be more focused

- Your liver will heal, which means your skin will repair itself and your digestive issues will slowly disappear
- You won't need to lie to your family about your drinking habits
- Everyone will respect you more

And if you need a role model to look up to as you try to quit the bottle, consider how many famous people have freed themselves from alcohol's liquor-stained grip to live an exceptional life of success. Here are a few of them, and here is what they had to say about quitting:

"I don't miss it. Now it's as if I had never had a drink in my life. At one point, I could never have conceived going out and not drinking, but as time goes on you lose the urge."
- Gerard Butler

"Simple as this, I quit drinking. It's really not that a big deal. It has no real bearing on anything else in my life. Your lifestyle changes at a certain age."
- Ben Affleck

"I still hang out in bars. I get something that looks like a drink so people don't know I'm not drinking, because I want to be accepted. So I have a tonic with lime and it

looks like a gin and tonic. People say things like 'if you hang out in a barbershop for long enough, you'll get a haircut. What? Shut up. People tell you stuff like that because they think you're going to fail, or sometimes they want you to so they can say 'I told you so'."
- Samuel L. Jackson

"Getting sober was one of the pivotal events in my life, along with becoming an actor and having a child. Of the three, finding my sobriety was the hardest thing."
- Gary Oldman

The Social Disease

Being addicted to alcohol has long been considered a disease of society that affects only those among us who:

- Are weak of will
- Lack basic self-control
- Have an addictive personality

But the reality is that we can class alcoholism as a medical disease. Consequently, it should be treated like all medical diseases - with medication and support.

So that you can liberate yourself from alcohol, you first need to learn how alcohol affects your nervous system and body. But more importantly, it's crucial you own up to having a problem. This is the first step towards finding a solution.

Quitting is possible, no matter how hard it is. It's doable. How To Set Yourself Free From Alcohol explains the steps you need to take that will help you to reclaim YOUR life.

CHAPTER 1: THE EFFECTS OF ALCOHOL

People have been consuming alcohol for almost as many years as there has been a civilization, with records suggesting the ancients were drinking it medicinally some ten-thousand years ago. Alcohol may still be an effective medicine, and in fact it does have some benefits to your health. When taken sensibly, alcohol can:

- Reduce your risk of cardiovascular disease
- Lengthen your life
- Boost your libido
- Reduce your risk of developing dementia

Drink too much, however, and it becomes a poison. It not only affects your body, but it also affects your mind. The way it destroys you both physically and mentally can wreck your social life, creating stress to you and those close to you. Moreover, alcohol doesn't discriminate but affects everyone, young and old, male or female.

The Factors That Determine The Way You React To Alcohol

Your Size

If you are a larger than average person, it follows that you have more blood, which allows you to contain alcohol and its effects more than someone smaller.

The Type Of Drink

Liquor contains more alcohol than a pint of beer, and will therefore have a bigger impact on you in a shorter period of time.

If you drink four glasses of whiskey during the same amount of time it takes your buddy to get through two pints of lager, you will get drunk much quicker - even though in terms of liquid, he has taken in more.

Glass Size

You might only be drinking a glass of wine, just like you did last night. But if you're drinking from a bigger glass this time, you will feel the effects of alcohol more.

How Long You Drink

The average adult is able to cope with around four drinks in six hours. If, however, you decide that today you're going to drink four beers in just two hours, the effects of the alcohol will be much more noticeable. You are not giving your body any chance to metabolize the alcohol.

How Much You Eat Before Drinking
It's common knowledge that if you head out on a night of drinking without eating a big meal beforehand, you will get drunk quicker.

How You Feel Emotionally
People respond differently to alcohol depending on how they feel emotionally. If you are happy and stress-free, it's unlikely that alcohol will trouble your mind. If, however, you are anxious and worried about something, alcohol can worsen your mental state considerably.

Your Body And Alcohol
Just a minor amount of alcohol in your body can be significant. Alcohol works quickly, and as soon as your bloodstream has absorbed it, it starts to affect your nervous system. As such, your long-term health is always at risk.

Your body consists of various network systems that rely on each other in order to keep you functioning optimally. Here is how too much alcohol can damage them:

The Circulatory System

If you drink too much alcohol, you can harm your heart. This is even the case if it's your first ever binge. For chronic drinkers, the effect is much worse. There are differences between how women and men handle their alcohol, with research showing that women put more strain on their heart than men when they drink. Complications arise more in women, too, and include heart attacks, heart failure, high blood pressure, and strokes.

The Excretory System

Drinking too much alcohol can cause your pancreas to unwittingly produce a number of poisonous chemicals. And once it does this, it is unable to perform its chief functions, such as regulating your insulin levels and disposing of waste products. Pancreatic inflammation can arise, which can eventually cause organ damage. Then there is the liver, which is also badly affected by too much alcohol in the body. Once it is inflamed, the liver is no longer able to carry out its function. This leads to your body being overrun with toxins, with jaundice, hepatitis and cirrhosis ailments.

The Nervous System

It doesn't take very long for alcohol to move through your body, and it can reach your nervous system and brain in almost zero time. When drunk, you might find that your speech becomes slurred, you have no control over your impulses, you've lost your balance, and you cannot recall something that just happened. Over time, alcohol can shrink your brain's frontal lobes. And once your nervous system is damaged, it can cause pain and unbearable numbness.

The Immune System
Alcohol compromises your immune system, leaving you vulnerable to infections and disease. There is a high rate of alcoholics suffering from pneumonia and cancer for this reason.

The Digestive System
Too much alcohol can have a damaging effect on the digestive system. Alcohol prevents your digestive tract from properly absorbing and using nutrients and vitamins, and it also stops it from regulating bacteria. Alcohol abuse can also cause tooth decay, mouth irritations, heartburn, gastritis, as well as internal bleeding.

The Reproductive System
Alcohol negatively impacts the human reproduction system of both genders in various ways. Symptoms in men may include infertility, diminished testicular functioning, as well as erectile dysfunction. Symptoms

in women can include infertility, a higher risk of breast cancer, as well as no menstruation.

It is advised that pregnant women abstain from drinking alcohol altogether, as it can cause miscarriage, stillbirth or a premature birth.

The Ways In Which Alcohol Is Eliminated From Your Body

The human body has two main ways in which it dispenses of alcohol:
- Oxidation
- Elimination
-

Oxidation

Oxidation plays the biggest role in the removal of alcohol from your body. Oxidation occurs when oxygen molecules combine with another substance's molecules, such as alcohol. Via oxidation, the human body is able to eliminate alcohol.

Each time you drink alcohol, the substance mixes with water and carbon dioxide in your liver. But because your liver cannot deal with more than a small amount of alcohol at any one time, most of it remains inside your bloodstream, where it then travels around the body. Consequently, it affects your tissues, cells and organs.

Alcohol only stops circulating when your liver is finally able to eliminate all of it, a process that takes some time.

Elimination
During elimination, the human body passes alcohol though your skin, lungs or kidneys.
Your kidneys eliminate alcohol via your urine. Your skin dispenses with it by sweating it out. Your lungs eliminate it by your breathing out. Each time you exhale, alcohol evaporates.

Many people who drink a lot of alcohol over a sustained period of time are just too unaware of the problems it is causing to their bodies. The impact is chronic, and just one binge can do damage that cannot be easily reversed. Understanding how alcohol affects you can help you to quit.

CHAPTER 2: SYMPTOMS AND SIGNS OF ALCOHOLISM

At which point do you know when your drinking has gone from moderate to full-blown dependence and abuse? First, you need to know the signs since it is crucial to understanding when it is time to take action.

It's fundamental that you know what alcohol abuse and alcoholism are. In many western cultures, drinking booze is just part and parcel of the culture. It's so common and expected that it is hard to know when someone is just being social and having a good time, and when they are actually reliant on alcohol. Making the distinction depends on how booze is impacting your life.

If you have ever found yourself in any of these situations, you may have a problem:

- You tell lies to obscure your alcohol habits
- You feel bad about your alcohol habits
- Alcohol makes you feel better about who you are
- You often drink more than you intended
- People have voiced concern over how much you drink
- You "black out" quite often when drinking

Alcoholism vs. Alcohol Abuse

There is a distinction between alcoholism and alcohol abuse. The former is a much more extreme form of abuse. Whereas we have a bit of control when we are abusing alcohol, we are physically and mentally dependent on alcohol when we are suffering from alcoholism. We cannot get though a day without it.

Symptoms And Signs Of Alcohol Abuse

Needing Booze To Relax Yourself

Alcohol abusers might crack open a bottle in the belief that it will help them unwind, de-stress and take care of their problems.

Continuing To Drink Even If It Is Ruining Your Relationship

If your loved ones - especially your partner - have told you they don't like you when you are drunk and want you to cut down, it's sensible to listen to them. If, however, you ignore their concerns and continue to drink regardless, you might be abusing alcohol.

Ignoring Your Responsibilities And Duties

We all have responsibilities and duties, and many of us will do whatever is necessary to make sure we maintain ours. Ordinarily, you probably do the same.

However, alcohol abuse can compel you to skip days at work and neglect your family or things you wouldn't normally even dream of doing.

Continuing To Drink In Spite Of The Physical Risks
You've already been given warning signs that drinking is putting you at harm, but you continue regardless.

Symptoms and Signs of Alcoholism

Tolerance
Perhaps the biggest warning sign that you have slipped into alcoholism is stronger tolerance levels. It now takes you a lot longer to get drunk. While you might think this is a good thing because it means you get to drink more, it's actually a sign that you are drinking too much.

Withdrawal
If you feel lousy in the morning to the extent that your body is actually shaking, you might find that the only way to make yourself feel better is by drinking alcohol. This, indeed, is the only way to remedy your symptoms, and it's a sign that your body is now so dependent on alcohol that it cannot function properly without it. In a sense, your cells have become alcohol cells, and until you consume more booze, your

symptoms of nausea, anxiety and trembling will continue.

Unable To Quit
Drinking is damaging your life, but you just cannot quit.

Can't Control How Much You Drink
You say you only want two or three beers tonight, but you end the night having drunk more than six or seven.

Alcohol Takes Precedence Over Important Things
You used to enjoy reading, seeing family and exercising. But all you have time for now is drinking.

You Know Damage Is Being Done, But You Still Drink
Your marriage is over, you've lost your job and you constantly feel ill. Despite your world falling apart around you, you still drink.

Slipping from abusing alcohol to full-blown alcoholism is easier than many people think. All it takes is one crucial incident in one's life, such as the death of a loved one, for a person to become an alcoholic. Although some would argue that alcohol is a reasonably acceptable coping mechanism in such circumstances, it doesn't take a lot for the coping mechanism to become destructive.

You Are In Denial

Alcohol abusers are generally in a perpetual state of denial. They will tell you they have their drinking under control, and they will rationalize everything they do. But you can see the pain they are going through.

Denial stops us from being honest with ourselves and those closest to us. Consequently, it can harm our relationships, careers, and especially our finances. How do you know if you are in denial about your drinking?

1) You shift the blame from yourself and onto other people.
2) You reassure your loved ones that it's no big deal.
3) You say nothing bad has ever happened as a result of your drinking. "Nobody died!"
4) You tell people you only have one or two drinks a night, even though the reality is that you average at least five.
Take a look at yourself and ask whether or not you do any of the above on a regular basis. Be honest with your answers.

CHAPTER 3: WITHDRAWAL FROM ALCOHOL

Withdrawal from alcohol has a set of very clear symptoms. When you stop drinking suddenly, or drastically reduce how much you drink, withdrawal symptoms will appear pretty quickly. Sometimes, they appear rapidly (within six hours), while sometimes they might appear gradually over a few days.

Symptoms include:
- Nausea
- Anxiety
- Seizures
- Hallucinations
- Fatigue
- High Blood Pressure
- Insomnia
- Nightmares
- Confusion
- Fever

As you can see, some symptoms are more severe than others, but all are crippling and do no feel good whatsoever. In fact, they feel so bad that you might find yourself quickly reaching for a drink.

If you drink a lot of booze each day, your body cannot help but become dependent on it. Also, your nervous system will become excited and irritable by all the alcohol constantly swimming around inside your body.

As such, it certainly notices when you suddenly take alcohol away from it. It can't cope, and the result is a whole bunch of withdrawal symptoms you must find a way of coping with.

And you really must, because withdrawal can actually be fatal if is:
a.) Extreme
b.) Mishandled

Diagnosing Withdrawal

If you feel that you are undergoing withdrawal from alcohol, it is imperative that you seek immediate medical assistance. You cannot get through this without professional help. Doing it by yourself will either result in grave consequences, or it might see you remedy the symptoms by drinking more alcohol. Your doctor will give you a thorough examination, and will ask you questions related to your drinking history, as well as any irregular sensations rippling through your body.

Treating Withdrawal

The way your symptoms are treated will depend on how severe they are. Usually, a milder case will be treated at your own home, but more severe symptoms will result in hospitalization. The doctors will want to make you as comfortable as possible, and they will also provide you with counseling to help you get through this.

If the doctor suggests a home treatment, it's essential that you invite a relative or friend over to keep track of how you're doing. If your condition worsens, you need someone there to call for help.

Your friend should also take you out for any medical tests you need to take, or any counseling appointments. But more than anything else, they should just be a friend to you - someone who you can talk to, and who can take your mind off things. This is a desperate situation, and you need someone by your side. It is practically impossible to overcome withdrawal alone.

More severe symptoms will be treated in a hospital, where a doctor can track you progress and handle any complications that might arise. Some of the medications you might be given include:

- Diazepam
- Lorazepam
- Clonazepam
- Alprazolam

You may also be given vitamin supplements.

The good news is that withdrawal from alcohol can be treated and overcome. As long as you don't touch alcohol and actually do what your doctors tell you to do, you will make a full recovery. Fatigue might linger for a while afterwards, but eventually even that symptom will disappear.

Prevention
How to avoid withdrawal? Stay away from booze.
If you are concerned that you might have a problem, see your doctor or call an alcohol counselor right away.

CHAPTER 4: THE JOURNEY TO RECOVERY

You can take your first huge step on the path to recovery right this minute. Why wait? It can begin now. If you're really committed about giving up alcohol and changing your life for the better, you can totally do it.

"But I might as well wait until I hit rock bottom." What?

Look. the road will be bumpy. There will be obstacles you have to meet head on and overcome. But you can only solve things in life by first admitting that there is a problem.

First Step - Make A Commitment To Yourself That You're Going to Quit Drinking

People who want to quit drinking tend to take things very slowly. It's not easy to find an alcoholic who has decided to fix their problem by going cold turkey. It very rarely works that way.

Denial is often the biggest obstacle at this point. Like with anything that seems difficult to do or even totally insurmountable, you might find yourself creating excuses for why you don't need to quit just yet. "My drinking isn't out of control that much."

"I don't feel that bad."
What separates those who quit drinking and go on to live a healthy and successful life from those who sit staring at a bottle for the next few years is that the first group of people took action.

It's one thing to say you have a problem, but it's another to take action. What are you going to do about your problem? Are you going to do something about it?

A useful thing to do at this point is to make two lists. The first will list the benefits you get if you keep drinking, while the second will list the benefits you'll get if you quit.

Here are some examples:

I should keep drinking because ...
1.) Drinking helps me to unwind after work
2.) Drinking loosens me up and I always have more fun
3.) Drinking helps me to avoid dealing with my issues

I should quit drinking because ...
1.) I'll have more time for my family and my passions in life. Oh, I could finish my novel ...
2.) My partner would be so grateful

3.) I would probably feel a lot healthier, mentally and physically

Also, consider what drinking is costing you:

Drinking is costing me ...
1.) Time, energy and money
2.) My relationship and some friendships
3.) My dignity
4.) My mental health

And how about this:

But If I stop drinking ...
1.) My friends who I drink with won't want to hang out anymore. They'll think I'm lame and that I've "changed"
2.) I'll have to confront the responsibilities I've avoided for so long
3.) How will I deal with my issues?

Second Step - Make Goals
Setting goals is not always so easy. I suggest that you use the SMART method of setting goals. Like this:

S - Be specific
M - Be measurable
A - Be attainable

R - Be realistic

T - Be time conscious

If you're not specific about your goals, you'll find it hard to stick to them. For example, being ultra vague by saying "I want to quit drinking" is just not enough. You need to get specific by writing down when you want to stop drinking.

Also, it's really important you're realistic about your goals. Setting yourself an impossible deadline to quit drinking by (such as tomorrow afternoon) is crazy and will not work.

Once you've set your goals, write down your strategy. This is basically how you plan on attaining your goals.

As part of your strategy, you might want to:
- Remove any alcohol or temptations to drink alcohol from your office and home.
- Tell your friends and family about your plans. Make yourself acceptable to them.
- Set boundaries. Tell people that they cannot drink in your house. Tell your friends you don't want to hang out in a pub. Suggest alternatives, such as a coffee house.
- If you have friends who pester you to drink, kick them out of your life. You don't need them.

- Create an alcohol diary, and write down each time you drink. Don't try to make your life look better than it is - record every drink
- When you do drink (or if), drink it slowly. Be mindful of how much you're putting into your body

Third Step - Put Your Safety Before Anything Else
If you think you can quit alcohol by yourself, then so be it. Do so. But if you do not think you can handle it, seek medical attention or ask a friend to move in with you for a while.

Fourth Step - Put A New Life Together
When people decide to quit alcohol, one of the first things they ask is, "But what am I gonna do instead? What am I gonna replace it with?"

It's a good question. Because alcohol was such a fundamental part of your life, you're now essentially building a new life. It's like when a pro athlete retires from the game. How on earth do they replace what they once had? It is easy to see why so many athletes fall into a spiral of depression upon retirement.

You can start a new life by:
1.) Finding yourself a support group, which consists of fellow recovering addicts. Find friends who you can relate to, and who are also trying to start a new life.

Involve yourself in a positive community who encourages you to stay motivated and do the right things.

2.) Take good care of yourself. Adopt a healthier diet. Exercise more, sleep more. This will improve your emotional wellbeing, reduce stress, and subsequently ensure that you don't miss alcohol. You will feel so much better you won't need a drink anymore.

3.) Find new things to do. Return to an old passion or find a new one. It's important that you stay busy so that your mind doesn't get a chance to wander back to alcohol. Spend some time volunteering or go on dates. Use your time productively. Read books, learn new things!

Fifth Step: Get Ready For The Cravings And Triggers

During the initial six months after cutting down (or cutting out) alcohol, you will experience some intense cravings. This is part of the process. You can manage cravings in the following ways:

1.) When you feel a craving coming on, instantly do an activity that will distract you. Something as simple as counting coins helps. You could also grab a newspaper and fill in a puzzle, go out for a run, or wash your car. It's all about directing your mind elsewhere.

2) Talk to someone you can trust when you feel a craving coming on. Phone up your sponsor, or ask someone out for coffee. Once you've asked them and they've agreed, you won't want to back out. You will go for a coffee instead of the pub.

3) Remind yourself how bad alcohol made you feel. Remind yourself what will happen if you have just one more sip. Remind yourself why you're doing this in the first place, and then remember how good life is right now.

4.) Practice mindfulness. Don't fight the cravings. Acknowledge them. Let them dance around in your mind, making all their noise. Then watch them leave.

Sixth Step - Get Support

As mentioned earlier, it's virtually impossible to get through this without your friends, family or a counselor. All recovering alcoholics need someone who will offer:

- Guidance
- Support
- Encouragement

- Comfort

Support can mean the difference between you getting through this successfully or relapsing. If you can't think of a way to get some support, here are a few suggestions:

1.) You could sign up to an alcohol recovery support group. If you do, you need to stay motivated to keep attending the meetings. These groups are very beneficial because they put you in direct contact with people who know exactly what you're going through. They can help you, you can help them, and you can make new friends.

2.) Your friends and family are ready to support you. All you need to do is ask. This is the hard bit, because it's normal to feel shame, guilt or embarrassment. But you have nothing to feel bad about. These are people who love you. They wont judge you, but they're ready to help you.

3.) Find ways of meeting new people. You could go volunteering, go on gallery tours, or attend general community events.

4.) Move to a new area. Sometimes, it's not just a case of finding support - sometimes it's a case of getting away from a circle that's very unsupportive. If you feel as though you could easily lapse into your old habits if you stay where you are (for example, perhaps you live across the road from a pub), it might be a good idea to move.

Seventh Step - Begin Your Treatment

As part of your treatment, you might want to seriously consider consulting a mental heath expert or professional. You might also want to consider getting yourself on an addiction program. This is because alcohol can lead to a wealth of mental disorders, including anxiety, depression and bipolar. As well as improving your physical condition, you will need to improve your mental health, too.

In conclusion to this treatment, it's important that you bear in mind that there is no magic bullet to treating alcoholism. What works for some might not work for you. As such, you need to take the time to find the right program for you.

When deciding on a treatment program, you should consider:
- Your lifestyle
- Your relationships
- Your health
- Your career

Once you have settled on a treatment program, you need to commit to it 100%.

CHAPTER 5: PREVENTING ALCOHOL RELAPSE

It takes a long time to recover from alcohol dependence, and you have to expect setbacks. Although you might go a week or two without a drink, don't be alarmed if you crack open a bottle again at some point. Although it isn't ideal, it happens. How you react to this is key. Do you see it as a personal failure and give up altogether? Or do you try again? The best way to avoid a relapse is to be proactive and remain diligent at all times. Keep your mind buzzing with thoughts, and keep yourself preoccupied with activities.

Give yourself something to do each day, but also be aware of potential triggers. Because you simply cannot hide away from the world, you need to be on your guard for triggers - because they will be out there.

WHAT CAUSES ALCOHOL RELAPSE?
There are a few things that can trigger a relapse, including:

Being Exposed To Alcohol
When we talk about exposure to alcohol, we talk about going to parties and evenings out where there will be alcohol. But you must also be wary of food that has

been cooked using alcohol, because this also counts as a trigger.

Stress

One of the major reasons people are driven to alcohol is stress. If you ask any alcoholic why they drink so much, it's very likely that they will say it helps them deal with the stresses and strains of living.

If stress is one of your triggers, it's important that you either find a way of avoiding stress, or learn about how to deal with stress effectively without alcohol. There are many ways to cope with stress without resorting to alcohol, including meditation, taking walks, deep breathing and so on.

Triggers Within The Environment

Environmental triggers include the people you hang around with, the restaurants you visit, the city you live in et cetera.

These ones can be especially hard to avoid. Lots of recovering alcoholics find that their social life changes hugely when they go out, because central to many of our shared activities is the pub.

You cannot avoid environmental triggers completely, which means you need to come up with a way of dealing with them.

HOW TO KNOW WHEN YOU ARE ON THE VERGE OF RELAPSE

Recovering addicts sometimes relapse, and there are certain warning signs that tell you and your family and friends that you are in danger of falling back into your old ways. Here are some of them:

You Reminisce Over The "Good Old Times"

Your friend is around your place tonight for a chat, and you find yourself smiling as you talk about old times.

"Remember that night when we both got so drunk that we ..."

Maybe you both have a good laugh as you bring up "fun" memories. But looking back fondly is only showing you one side of the story. You're editing out all the bad stuff that happened when you drank, and focusing on the highlights reel. And this is dangerous.

Wondering If You Could Drink Just To Be Social

Your friends are having a few drinks tonight, and you wonder how bad it would be if you popped out for "one or two." You don't need to go mad like you used to, but could instead have a few "quiet ones" before returning home. After all, it's rude not to be social, right? However, just a single drink can bring back the dark days.

Seeing Your Old Drinking Pals Again
When you first quit alcohol, you cut your old drinking buddies out of your life. But they've crept back in, and seeing their faces is making you wonder whether or not one drink really would kill you.

You Feel Forlorn
Recovering alcoholics who start to feel sad, depressed or even lonely could be on the short road to a full-blown relapse. Negative emotions like this are hard to handle when we're feeling especially vulnerable. But you have to ride with them rather than try to fight or escape them. They will pass.

You Withdraw From Your Support Group
Withdrawing from your support group is a very dangerous move. You need them more than you realize, and saying that you don't is not the thing to do right now.

You've Lost Interest In Your Hobbies
If nothing seems of interest to you anymore, negative thoughts may soon start to creep in. Recovering alcoholics need to stay busy, but if you can't bring yourself to do anything at all, the boredom might signal a relapse.

No Longer Believing In Your Recovery Program

If you think your recovery program just isn't working, you should consider what this means. The likelihood is that you're more frustrated by the fact that it's trying to keep you sober. Resenting your recovery program is not ideal.

HOW TO AVOID A RELAPSE

Go To A Support Group

One of the most popular support groups for alcoholics is Alcoholics Anonymous (AA), which provides addicts with a structure to help them stay sober. It offers both support and encouragement to the individual.

AA is built on a one-day-at-a-time philosophy, which basically means that you should cut out all thoughts you have about the future and focus only on getting to the end of each day.

AA members have meetings, where they get together and talk about how they reached the point of where they are. By sharing stories about their recovery, they encourage and inspire others. Each member has something to teach everybody else, such as how to handle triggers.

AA is also built around a twelve-step program that consists of a list of twelve ideas that helps each member to stay sober. The program also offers its members a sponsor who helps them to make a full recovery from their addiction.

Therapy

Therapy can help you to deal with setbacks and possible triggers. It arms you with the skills needed to avoid a relapse.

Therapy is particularly good for recovering alcoholics who give in easily to social pressure, and who are not sure how they will handle environmental triggers. Being proactive and seeking out a therapist could be the main thing that stops you from relapsing.

Medication

A recovering addict can take prescription drugs that will stop a relapse from occurring. Disulfiram, for example, trains both your mind and body so that it recognizes how drinking negatively impacts you. It will also dispel the myth that drinking is somehow a positive thing.

You should avoid alcohol if you take Disulfiram. Otherwise, you will experience nasty side effects, such as vomiting, confusion and headaches.

Any medication you do take must be prescribed first of all by a doctor, and should not be your sole defense against a relapse. Medication by itself is just not enough, and you will need to combine it with either therapy or a support group.

CONCLUSION

Thank you buying this book and taking the time to read it. I'm pleased you made it to the end.
I hope now that you are ready to quit drinking. Better still, perhaps you have already started and are on your way to a cleaner, healthier, better you.

Be ruthless about this. Take no prisoners. You can be so much more if you quit alcohol. Your life will improve in a million ways. There is still so much time for you to live the life you've always wanted.

As mentioned in the book, it's all about taking action and making that commitment to being sober. Do it today. Take action, not just for yourself but also for your loved ones.

Good luck.

THANKS FOR READING

We really hope you enjoyed this book. If you found this material helpful feel free to share it with friends. You can also help others find it by leaving a review where you purchased the book. Your feedback will help us continue to write books you love.

The Smart Reads library is growing by the day! Make sure and check out the other wonderful books in our catalog. We would love to hear which books are your favorite.

Visit:

www.smartreads.co/freebooks

to receive Smart Reads books for FREE

Check us out on Instagram:

www.instagram.com/smart_readers

@smart_readers

Don't forget your 2 FREE audiobooks.
Use this link www.audibletrial.com/Travis to claim
your 2 FREE Books.

SMART READS ORIGINS

Smart Reads was born out of the desire to find the best information fast without having to wade through the sheer volume of fluff available online. Smart Reads combs through massive amounts of knowledge compiles the best into quick to read books on a variety of subjects.

We consider ourselves Smart Readers, not dummies. We know reading is smart. We're self taught. We like to learn a TON about a WIDE variety of topics. We have developed a love for books and we find intelligence attractive.

We found that each new topic we tried to learn about started with the challenge of finding the pieces of the puzzle that mattered most. It becomes a treasure hunt rather than an education.

Smart Reads wants to find the best of the best information for you. To condense it into a package that you can consume in an hour or less. So you can read more books about more topics in less time.

OUR MISSION

Smart Reads aims to accelerate the availability of useful information and will publish a high quality book on every major topic on amazon.

Smart Reads hopes to remove barriers to sharing by taking the copyright off everything we publish and donating it to the public domain. We hope other publishers and authors will follow our example.

Our goal is to donate $1,000,000 or more by 2020 to build over 2,000 schools by giving 5% of our net profit to Pencils of Promise.

We want to restore forests around the globe by planting a tree for every 10 physical books we sell and hope to plant over 100,000 trees by 2020.

Doesn't it feel good knowing that by educating yourself you are helping the world be a better place? We think so too...

Thanks for helping us help the world. You Smart Reader you...

Travis and the Smart Reads Team

WHY I STARTED SMART READS

Every time I wanted to learn about something new I'd have to buy 20 books on the topic and spend way too long sorting through them and reading them all until I arrived at the big picture. Until I had enough perspectives to know who was just guessing, who was uninformed and who had stumbled upon something remarkable.

I wished someone else could just go in and figure that out for me and tell me what matters. That's how smart reads was born. I want smart reads to be a company that does all that research up front. Sorts through all the content that is available on each topic and pulls out the most up to date complete understanding, then have people smarter than me package the best wisdom in an easy to understand way in the least amount of words possible.

For example, I got a new puppy so I wanted to learn about dog training. I bought 14 different books about dog training and by the time I got through the first 5 and finally started getting the big picture on the best way to train my puppy she had grown up into a dog.

Yeah she's well behaved. She doesn't poop in the house. I can get her to sit and come when I call. But what if someone else went in and read all those books for me, found the underlying themes and picked out the best information that would give me the big picture and get me right to the point. And I'd only have to read one book instead of 15.

That would be amazing. I would save time. And maybe my dog would be rolling over, cleaning up after my kids and doing the dishes by now. That my friend, is the reason I started smart reads. Because I wanted a company I can trust to deliver me the best information in an easy to understand way that I can digest in under an hour. Because dog training is one of many subjects I want to master.

The quicker I can learn a wide variety of topics the sooner that information can begin playing a role in shaping my future. And none of us knows how long that future will be. So why not do everything we can to make the best of it and consume a ton of knowledge. And I figured all the better if I can also make a positive difference in the world.

That's why we're also building schools, planting trees and challenging ideas about copyright's place in today's world. Because as a company we have to be doing everything we can to support the ecosystem that gives us all these beautiful places to read our books. Thanks for reading.

Travis

Customers Who Bought This
Customers Who Bought This Book
Also Bought

Dealing With Anxiety: Modern Techniques for an Age Old Condition

Success Principles: Techniques for Positive Thinking, Self Love and Developing a Powerful

Meditation Magic: Free Yourself from Worry, Depression, Stress and Anxiety

Develop Self-Discipline: Daily Habit to Make Self Confidence and Will Power Automatic

Natural Ways of Boosting Testosterone: How to Bulk Up and Put Your Sex Drive in Overdrive

Reinvent Yourself: Become Instantly Likable, Captivate Anyone in Seconds and Always Know What To Say

Unlocking Potential - Master the Laws of Leadership